The Easy Ketogenic Recipe Guide

Amazing Recipes to Discover the Benefits of Ketogenic Diet and Stay Fit

Lauren Loose

2

Contents

Mashed Potatoes and Parsnips

Preparation Time: 10 minutes

Cooking Time: 20 minutes

Serving: 4-6

Ingredients:

- 2 cups water
- 2 lbs. Yukon gold potatoes, peeled and cubed
- ¾ lb. parsnips, cut into 1-inch thick pieces
- 1 tsp. sea salt
- 1 tsp. ground black pepper
- 5 tbsp. half and half
- 2 tbsp. butter, melted

Directions:

1. Prepare the Instant Pot by adding the water to the pot and placing the steamer basket in it. Put the potatoes and parsnips in the basket.
2. Close and lock the lid. Select MANUAL and cook at HIGH pressure for 7 minutes. When the timer goes off, use a Quick Release. Carefully open the lid. Transfer the potatoes and parsnips to the bowl. Season with salt and pepper. Stir well.

3. Using a potato masher or electric beater, slowly blend half and half and butter into vegetables until smooth and creamy. Serve warm.

Nutrition:

226.4 Calories

6.1g Total Fat

18.8mg Cholesterol

34.4mg Sodium

Mashed Potatoes with Garlic and Rosemary

Preparation Time: 10 minutes

Cooking Time: 25 minutes

Serving: 4-6

Ingredients:

- 6 large potatoes, peeled and cubed
- 3 cloves garlic
- 1 sprig rosemary
- 1 cup chicken broth
- ¼ cup milk
- 2 tbsp. butter
- Salt to taste

Directions:

1. In the Instant pot, combine the potatoes, garlic, rosemary, and broth. Stir well. Close and lock the lid. Select MANUAL and cook at HIGH pressure for 15 minutes.
2. Once timer goes off, use a Quick Release. Carefully unlock the lid. Drain the potatoes. Using a potato masher or electric beater, slowly blend milk and butter into potatoes until smooth and creamy.
3. Season with salt and serve.

Nutrition:

130.7 Calories

4g Total Fat

164.7mg Sodium

Scalloped Potatoes

Preparation Time: 10 minutes

Cooking Time: 25 minutes

Serving: 2-4

Ingredients:

- 6 medium potatoes, peeled and thinly-sliced
- 1 tbsp. chives, chopped
- ½ tsp. kosher salt
- ¼ tsp. ground black pepper
- 1 cup chicken broth
- 1/3 cup sour cream
- 1/3 cup milk
- 2 tbsp. potato starch
- ¼ tsp. paprika

Directions:

1. Add the potatoes, chives, salt and pepper to the Instant Pot. Pour in the broth and stir. Close and lock the lid.
2. Select MANUAL and cook at HIGH pressure for 5 minutes. Once pressure cooking is complete, select CANCEL and use a Quick Release. Carefully unlock the lid.

3. Transfer the potatoes to the baking sheet. Preheat the oven to broil. In the Instant Pot, combine the remaining liquid, sour cream, milk, and potato starch.

4. Select SAUTÉ and cook the mixture for 1 minute, until thickened. Pour the mixture over the potatoes and stir. Sprinkle with paprika and place under the broiler for 3 to 5 minutes for a browned top.

Nutrition:

20g Carbohydrates

12g Fat

6g Protein

Garlic Roasted Potatoes

Preparation Time: 15 minutes

Cooking Time: 30 minutes

Serving: 4-6

Ingredients:

- 5 tbsp. vegetable oil
- 5 cloves garlic
- 2 lbs. baby potatoes
- 1 rosemary spring
- ½ cup stock
- Salt and ground black pepper to taste

Directions:

1. Select the SAUTÉ setting on the Instant Pot and heat the oil. Add the garlic, potatoes and rosemary. Cook, stirring occasionally, for 10 minutes or until the potatoes start to brown.

2. Using a fork, pierce the middle of each potato. Pour in the stock. Season with salt and pepper. Stir well. Press the CANCEL key to stop the SAUTÉ function.

3. Close and lock the lid. Select MANUAL and cook at HIGH pressure for 7 minutes. When the timer beeps, use a Quick Release. Carefully unlock the lid. Serve.

Nutrition:

180 Calories

8.6g Total Fats

501mg Sodium

2.7g Protein

Autumn Potatoes Salad

Preparation Time: 10 minutes

Cooking Time: 25 minutes

Serving: 4-6

Ingredients:

- 1½ cups water
- 4 eggs
- 6 medium potatoes, peeled and cut into 1½ inch cubes
- 1 tbsp. dill pickle juice
- 1 cup homemade mayonnaise
- 2 tbsp. parsley, finely chopped
- ¼ cup onion, finely chopped
- 1 tbsp. mustard
- Salt and ground black pepper to taste

Directions:

1. Pour the water into the Instant Pot and insert a steamer basket. Place the eggs and potatoes in the basket. Select MANUAL and cook at HIGH pressure for 5 minutes.
2. When the timer goes off, use a Quick Release. Carefully open the lid. Transfer the eggs to the bowl of cold water. Wait 2-3 minutes.

3. In another bowl, combine the dill pickle juice, mayo, parsley, onion, and mustard. Mix well. Add the potatoes and gently stir to coat with the sauce. Peel eggs, chop and add to the salad. Stir well.

4. Season with salt and pepper, stir and serve.

Nutrition:

180 Calories

17g Carbohydrates

11g Fat

3g Protein

Red Potato and Bacon Salad

Preparation Time: 10 minutes

Cooking Time: 15 minutes

Serving: 6-8

Ingredients:

- 1½ cups water
- 6 eggs
- 3 lbs. red potatoes, peeled and cut into 1½ inch cubes
- 2 cups mayonnaise
- ½ lb. cooked bacon, sliced into 1-inch thick pieces
- 2 celery stalks, chopped
- 1 bunch green onions
- Salt and ground black pepper to taste

Directions:

1. Pour the water into the Instant Pot and insert a steamer basket. Place the eggs and potatoes in the basket.
2. Select MANUAL and cook at HIGH pressure for 5 minutes. When the timer goes off, use a Quick Release. Carefully open the lid.
3. Transfer the eggs to the bowl of cold water. Wait 2-3 minutes. In the large bowl, combine

the cooked potatoes, mayonnaise, bacon, celery and green onion. Peel eggs, chop and add to the salad. Stir well.

4. Season with salt and pepper, stir and serve.

Nutrition:

240.8 Calories

6.2g Sodium

5.3g Protein

Red Potato with Cheese

Preparation Time: 20 minutes

Cooking Time: 40 minutes

Serving: 2-4

Ingredients:

- 1 tbsp. butter
- 1 lb. red potatoes, cut into 1-inch cubes
- 1 cup chicken broth
- 1 tsp. dried rosemary
- 1 tsp. dried oregano
- 1 tsp. dried parsley
- ¼ tsp. salt
- ½ cup parmesan cheese, shredded

Directions:

1. Add the butter to the Instant Pot and select SAUTÉ. Once the butter has melted, add the potatoes. Stir until well coated and sauté for 5 minutes. Add the broth, rosemary, oregano, and parsley. Close and lock the lid.

2. Press the CANCEL button to reset the cooking program, then press the MANUAL button and set the cooking time for 5 minutes at HIGH pressure. When the timer beeps, use a Natural Release for 10 minutes. Uncover the pot.

3. Season with salt and cheese and gently stir. Serve.

Nutrition:

196.3 Calories

3.7g Total Fat

2.3g Fiber

Baked Radish Snack

Preparation Time: 8 minutes

Cooking Time: 22 minutes

Servings: 2

Ingredients:

- 8 oz. red radishes, washed and trimmed
- 2 Tbsp. olive oil
- 2 Tbsp. unsalted butter
- 1 clove garlic, diced
- 1 tsp. lemon juice
- ¼ tsp. oregano, dried
- Salt and pepper, to taste
- 1 pinch parsley

Direction

1. Place the halved or quartered radishes into a separate bowl. Drizzle over the olive oil and add oregano. Stir gently.
2. Put the radish on the baking sheet and place it in the oven (preheated to 450°F).
3. Bake for 18-22 minutes. Mix occasionally.
4. Melt the butter in a saucepan. Add garlic and cook for about 3-5 minutes.

5. Remove your roasted radishes from the oven, sprinkle them with lemon juice and top with the butter mix.

Nutrition:

17g Fat

1g Protein

164 Calories

Boiled Asparagus with
Sliced Lemon

Preparation Time: 5 minutes

Cooking Time: 7 minutes

Servings: 1

Ingredients:

- 10 large beans asparagus
- 3 Tbsp. avocado oil
- ¼ Tbsp. lemon juice
- 2-3 pieces lemon
- ¼ cup water
- ½ tsp. salt

Directions:

1. Place the asparagus in a pot of water. Boil for about 5-7 minutes.
2. Take the asparagus out of the pot. Sprinkle with lemon juice, avocado oil, and salt. Serve with the pieces of lemon.

Nutrition:

43g Fat

4.7g Protein

447 Calories

Stuffed Eggs with Bacon-Avocado Filling

Preparation Time: 10 minutes

Cooking Time: 10 minutes

Servings: 1

Ingredients:

- 2 eggs, boiled and halved
- 1 Tbsp. mayonnaise
- ¼ tsp. mustard
- 1/8 lemon, squeezed
- ¼ tsp. garlic powder
- 1/8 tsp. salt
- 1/8 tsp. smoked paprika
- ¼ avocado
- 16 small pieces bacon

Direction:

1. Fry the bacon for 3 minutes in a pan. Add the avocado and fry for an additional 3 minutes (lower heat).
2. Combine the mayonnaise, mustard, lemon, garlic powder, and salt in a separate bowl. Stir well.
3. Scoop out yolk from the halved eggs and fill the egg halves with the mayonnaise mix. Top with the bacon-avocado filling.

Nutrition:

30g Fat

16g Protein

342 Calories

Crab Cakes with Almond Flour

Preparation Time: 1 hour 10 minutes

Cooking time: 15 minutes

Servings: 4

Ingredients:

- 8 oz. fresh crab meat, shells removed
- 1 Tbsp. garlic, minced
- ¼ cup parsley, chopped
- 1 egg, slightly beaten
- 1 Tbsp. avocado oil mayonnaise
- 1 Tbsp. mustard
- ½ tsp. kosher salt
- ½ tsp. dried thyme
- 1/8 tsp. cayenne pepper
- ½ cup almond flour
- 2 Tbsp. butter, for frying

Direction:

1. In a separate bowl, combine the crabmeat, garlic, parsley, egg, mayonnaise, mustard, kosher salt, thyme, cayenne pepper, and almond flour. Stir well. Form 4 cakes and place them into a fridge for 1 hour.
2. Melt the butter in the pan and put in your crab cakes. Fry for 6 minutes per side.

Nutrition:

17g Fat

13g Protein

219 Calories

Spicy Zucchini Chips

Preparation Time: 5 minutes

Cooking Time: 5 minutes

Servings: 4

Ingredients:

- 1 large zucchini, finely sliced
- 1 Tbsp. taco seasoning
- Coconut oil, for frying
- Salt to taste

Direction:

1. Wet the zucchini slices and sprinkle them with salt. Leave for 5 minutes.
2. Put the sliced zucchini into the frying pan and fry for 1-3 minutes on each side.
3. Top the fried slices with taco seasoning and enjoy your snack.

Nutrition:

6.12g Fat

0.2g Protein

164 Calories

Cheesy Broccoli with Chives

Preparation Time: 10 minutes

Cooking Time: 15 minutes

Servings: 4

Ingredients:

- 2 cups Shredded cheddar cheese
- 1 Broccoli head; florets separated
- 1 tbsp. Chopped chives
- 4 cups Chicken stock
- 1 cup Coconut cream
- What you'll need from the store cupboard:
- ¼ tsp. Garlic powder
- A pinch of salt and white pepper

Directions:

1. Mix the chives, stock, broccoli florets, salt, and white pepper, and garlic powder in the instant pot, seal the lid to cook for 10 minutes at high pressure.
2. Natural release the pressure for 10 minutes and change the pot setting to 'Sauté.' Mix in the cream and cheese and blend with a dipping blender then let it cook for 5 minutes.
3. Share into bowls and serve.

Nutrition:

376 Calories

33.5g fat

16.2g protein

1.4g fiber

Brussels Sprouts Cream

Preparation Time: 10 minutes

Cooking Time: 20 minutes

Servings: 4

Ingredients:

- 1 tbsp. Chopped chives
- 1 cup Chicken stock
- 2 Chopped shallots
- 1 lb. Halved Brussels sprouts
- 1 cup Coconut cream
- A pinch of salt and black pepper
- 1 tbsp. Olive oil

Directions:

1. Press 'Sauté' on the instant pot and add the olive oil. When it is hot, reduce the shallots in the oil for 5 minutes.
2. Mix in the cream, stock, Brussels sprouts, salt, and pepper then seal the lid to cook for 20 minutes at high pressure.
3. Quick-release the pressure for 5 minutes, sprinkle the chives into the mix and stir the stew, share into bowls and serve.

Nutrition:

220 Calories

16.7g fat

5.4g protein

Nutmeg Spiced Endives

Preparation Time: 10 minutes

Cooking Time: 10 minutes

Servings: 4

Ingredients:

- 4 (trimmed and halved) Endives
- 1 cup Water
- 1 tsp. (ground) Nutmeg
- 1 tbsp. (chopped) Chives
- 2 tbsp. Olive oil
- Salt and black pepper to the taste

Directions:

1. Pour water into the Instant Pot and place the steamer basket over it. Place endives in this steamer basket.
2. Seal the pot's lid and cook for 10 minutes on manual mode at High. Allow the pressure to release in 10 minutes naturally then remove the lid. Toss them with salt, pepper, nutmeg, oil and chives.
3. Serve fresh and enjoy.

Nutrition:

63 Calories

7.2g Total Fat

0.1g Protein

0.1g. Fiber

Cabbage Radish Medley

Preparation Time: 10 minutes

Cooking Time: 15 minutes,

Servings: 4

Ingredients:

- 1 (shredded) Red cabbage head
- 2 tbsp. Veggie stock
- 1 cup (sliced) Radish
- 1 tbsp. Coconut amino
- ½ inch (grated) Ginger
- 1 tbsp. Olive oil
- 3 (minced) Garlic cloves

Directions:

1. Let your Instant Pot preheat on Sauté mode. Add oil, ginger, and garlic to the pot. Sauté for 3 minutes, then stir in remaining ingredients.
2. Seal the lid pot's lid and cook for 12 minutes on manual high settings. Allow the pressure to release naturally in 10 minutes. Serve warm and fresh.

Nutrition:

83 Calories

4.4g Total Fat

2.6g Protein

2.1g. Fiber

Saucy Passata Brussels Sprouts

Preparation Time: 10 minutes

Cooking Time: 10 minutes,

Servings: 4

Ingredients:

- 1-pound (halved) Brussels sprouts
- ¼ cup Chicken stock
- 1 tbsp. (chopped) Green onions
- 1 tbsp. (chopped) Chives
- 1 cup Tomato passata

Directions:

1. Add sprouts, stock, salt, black pepper, passata, chives, olive oil and green onions to the Instant Pot.
2. Seal the lid of the pot and cook for 10 minutes on Manual mode at High. Allow the pressure to release naturally in 10 minutes.
3. Serve fresh.

Nutrition:

112 Calories

7.5g Total Fat

4g Protein

2.4g. Fiber

Cheesy Broccoli Bites

Preparation Time: 15 minutes

Cooking Time: 10 minutes

Servings: 4

Ingredients:

- 1-pound Broccoli florets
- ½ cup Veggie stock
- 2 (chopped) Shallots
- 1 cup (shredded) Mozzarella cheese
- 1 tbsp. (chopped) Cilantro

Directions:

1. Let your Instant pot preheat on Sauté mode. Add oil and shallots to the pot and stir cook for 2 minutes. Stir in remaining ingredients except for the mozzarella cheese.

2. Mix well then top the mixture with mozzarella cheese. Seal the lid of the pot and cook for 8 minutes on manual mode at High. Allow the pressure to release naturally for 10 minutes. Serve fresh and enjoy.

Nutrition:

149 Calories

12.1g Total Fat

5.2g Protein

3g Fiber

Balsamic Mushrooms

Preparation Time: 10 minutes

Cooking Time: 15 minutes,

Servings: 4

Ingredients:

- 1 pound (sliced) White mushrooms
- ¼ cup Chicken stock
- 1 cup (sliced) Radishes
- 1 tbsp. (chopped) Parsley
- What you'll need from the store cupboard:
- 2 tbsp. Avocado oil
- 2 tbsp. Balsamic vinegar
- a pinch Salt and black pepper

Directions:

1. Let your Instant Pot preheat on Sauté mode. Add oil and mushrooms to sauté for 5 minutes. Stir in remaining ingredients and mix well Seal the pot's lid and cook for 10 minutes on manual mode at High.
2. Allow the pressure to release in 10 minutes then remove the lid. Serve fresh and enjoy.

Nutrition:

41 Calories

4.3g Total Fat

3.9g Protein

1.9g. Fiber

Balsamic Glazed Spinach

Preparation Time: 5 minutes

Cooking Time: 12 minutes,

Servings: 4

Ingredients:

- ¼ cup Veggie stock
- 1 and ½ pound Baby spinach
- 1 tbsp. (chopped) Walnuts
- 1 tbsp. (chopped) Chives
- 1 tbsp. Balsamic vinegar

Directions:

1. Add spinach along with all the ingredients to the Instant Pot. Seal the pot's lid and cook for 7 minutes on manual mode at High.
2. Allow the pressure to release in 5 minutes then remove the lid. Serve fresh and enjoy.

Nutrition:

13 Calories

1.2g Total Fat:

0.5g Protein

0.2g. Fiber

Tangy White Mushrooms

Preparation Time: 10 minutes

Cooking Time: 25 minutes

Servings: 4

Ingredients:

- 1 and ½ pound (sliced) White mushrooms
- 1 cup Veggie stock
- 1 tbsp. (chopped) Dill
- 1 tbsp. (chopped) Rosemary
- 1 tbsp. Avocado oil
- 1 tbsp. Sweet paprika
- a pinch Salt and black pepper

Directions:

1. Let your Instant Pot preheat on Sauté mode. Add oil and mushrooms, to sauté for 5 minutes. Stir in remaining ingredients and mix well

2. Seal the pot's lid and cook for 10 minutes on manual mode at High. Allow the pressure to release in 10 minutes then remove the lid. Serve fresh and enjoy.

Nutrition:

14 Calories

2.3g Total Fat

0.5g Protein

1.3g. Fiber

Creamy Coconut Spinach

Preparation Time: 5 minutes

Cooking Time: 12 minutes

Servings: 4

Ingredients:

- 1 and ½ lbs. Baby spinach
- 1 tbsp. (chopped) Cilantro
- ¼ cup Coconut cream
- 1 tbsp. Chili powder
- Salt and black pepper

Directions:

1. Add spinach along with all the remaining ingredients to the Instant Pot. Seal the pot's lid and cook for 7 minutes on manual mode at High.
2. Allow the pressure to release in 5 minutes then remove the lid. Serve fresh and enjoy.

Nutrition:

41 Calories

3.9g Total Fat

0.6g Protein

1g. Fiber

Chili Eggplant Luncheon

Preparation Time: 10 minutes

Cooking Time: 15 minutes

Servings: 4

Ingredients:

- 1 big (cubed) Eggplant
- 1-pound (halved) Collard greens
- ½ cup Chicken stock
- 1 tbsp. (chopped) Cilantro
- 4 (chopped) Green onions
- 2 tbsp. Avocado oil
- 2 tsp. Chili paste

Directions:

1. Let your Instant Pot preheat on Sauté mode. Add oil, eggplants, and spring onions to sauté for 4 minutes. Stir in remaining ingredients and mix well.

2. Seal the pot's lid and cook for 10 minutes on manual mode at High. Allow the pressure to release in 10 minutes then remove the lid. Serve fresh and enjoy.

Nutrition:

84 Calories

2.4g Total Fat

4.2g Protein

2g. Fiber:

Easy Italian Asparagus

Preparation Time: 5 minutes

Cooking Time: 3 minutes

Servings: 4

Ingredients:

- 1 cup Water
- 1-pound (trimmed) Asparagus
- 1 tbsp. (chopped) Cilantro
- 1 tbsp. Lemon juice
- 1 tsp. Olive oil
- ½ tbsp. Italian seasoning
- a pinch Salt and black pepper

Directions:

1. Pour water into the Instant Pot and place steamer basket over it. Place asparagus in the steamer basket. Seal the pot's lid and cook for 4 minutes on manual mode at High.

2. Allow the pressure to release in 4 minutes naturally then remove the lid. Toss the asparagus with all other ingredients in a platter. Serve fresh and enjoy.

Nutrition:

39 Calories

2.1g Total Fat

2.5g Protein

1.1g. Fiber

White Mushrooms and Chard Mix

Preparation Time: 10 minutes

Cooking Time: 12 minutes,

Servings: 4

Ingredients:

- 1 pound (sliced) White mushrooms
- 1 red (roughly chopped) Chard bunch
- ¼ cup Chicken stock
- 3 tbsp. (chopped) Parsley
- 2 tbsp. Olive oil
- 1 tsp. Garlic powder
- a pinch Salt and black pepper

Directions:

1. Let your Instant Pot preheat on Sauté mode. Add oil and mushrooms to sauté for 2 minutes.
2. Stir in remaining ingredients and mix well. Seal the pot's lid and cook for 10 minutes on manual mode at High.
3. Allow the pressure to release in 10 minutes then remove the lid. Serve fresh and enjoy.

Nutrition:

88 Calories

7.4g Total Fat

3.8g Protein

1.3g. Fiber

Creamy Coconut Cauliflower

Preparation Time: 10 minutes

Cooking Time: 15 minutes

Servings: 4

Ingredients:

- 1-pound Cauliflower florets
- 1 cup (chopped) Red onion
- ¼ cup Chicken stock
- 1 cup Coconut cream
- 2 tbsp. Balsamic vinegar
- a pinch Salt and black pepper

Directions:

1. Add cauliflower along with remaining ingredients to the Instant Pot. Seal the pot's lid and cook for 15 minutes on manual mode at High. Allow the pressure to release in 10 minutes then remove the lid. Serve fresh and enjoy.

Nutrition:

180 Calories

14.5g Total Fat

4g Protein

4.5g. Fiber

Parmesan Cream Green Beans

Preparation Time: 10 minutes

Cooking Time: 15 minutes

Servings: 4

Ingredients:

- 10 oz. (trimmed and halved) Green beans
- 1/3 cup (grated) Parmesan
- 2 oz. Cream cheese
- 1 tbsp. (chopped) Dill
- 1/3 cup Coconut cream
- A pinch Salt and black pepper

Directions:

1. Add green beans, cream cheese and all the ingredients to the Instant Pot. Seal the pot's lid and cook for 15 minutes on manual mode at High.
2. Allow the pressure to release in 10 minutes then remove the lid. Serve fresh and enjoy.

Nutrition:

119 Calories

9.8g Total Fat

3g Protein

3g. Fiber

Flaxseed Pumpkin Muffins

Preparation Time: 10 minutes

Cooking Time: 15 minutes

Servings: 18

Ingredients

- ¼ cup sunflower seed butter
- ¾ cup pumpkin puree
- 2 tablespoons flaxseed meal
- ¼ cup coconut flour
- ½ cup erythritol
- ½ teaspoon nutmeg, ground
- 1 teaspoon cinnamon, ground
- ½ teaspoon baking soda
- 1 egg
- ½ teaspoon baking powder
- A pinch of salt

Directions

1. In a bowl, scourge butter with pumpkin puree and egg and blend well. Mix in flaxseed meal, coconut flour, erythritol, baking soda, baking powder, nutmeg, cinnamon and a pinch of salt and stir well.

2. Scoop into a greased muffin pan, situate in the oven at 350 degrees F and bake for 15 minutes. Allow to cool down and serve!

Nutrition:

65 Calories

2.82g Protein

5.42g Fat

Marinated Eggs

Preparation Time: 87 minutes

Cooking Time: 7 minutes

Servings: 4

Ingredients

- 6 eggs
- 1 and ¼ cups water
- ¼ cup unsweetened rice vinegar
- 2 tablespoons coconut aminos
- Salt and black pepper to the taste
- 2 garlic cloves, minced
- 1 teaspoon stevia
- 4 ounces cream cheese
- 1 tablespoon chives, chopped

Directions

1. Situate eggs in a pot, add water to cover, bring to a boil over medium heat, cover and cook for 7 minutes. Soak eggs with cold water and leave them aside to cool down. In a bowl, stir 1 cup water with coconut aminos, vinegar, stevia and garlic and whisk well.
2. Fill eggs in this mix, cover with a kitchen towel and leave them aside for 2 hours rotating from time to time. Peel eggs, slice into 2 and put egg

yolks in a bowl. Stir in ¼ cup water, cream cheese, salt, pepper and chives.

3. Place egg whites with this mix and serve them. Enjoy!

Nutrition:

289 Calories

15.86g Protein

22.6g Fat

Sausage and Cheese Dip

Preparation Time: 10 minutes

Cooking Time: 80 minutes

Servings: 28

Ingredients

- 8 ounces cream cheese
- A pinch of salt and black pepper
- 16 ounces sour cream
- 8 ounces pepper jack cheese, chopped
- 15 ounces canned tomatoes mixed with habaneros
- 1-pound Italian sausage, ground
- ¼ cup green onions, chopped

Directions

1. Preheat pan over medium heat, add sausage, stir and cook until it browns. Cook tomatoes mix for 4 minutes more.
2. Sprinkle pinch of salt, pepper and the green onions, stir and cook for 4 minutes. Spread pepper jack cheese on the bottom of your slow cooker.
3. Mix in cream cheese, sausage mix and sour cream, cover and cook on High for 2 hours.

Uncover your slow cooker, stir dip, transfer to a bowl and serve. Enjoy!

Nutrition:

132 Calories

6.79g Protein

9.58g Fat

Tasty Onion and
Cauliflower Dip

Preparation Time: 60 minutes

Cooking Time: 30 minutes

Servings: 24

Ingredients

- 1 and ½ cups chicken stock
- 1 cauliflower head, florets separated
- ¼ cup mayonnaise
- ½ cup yellow onion, chopped
- ¾ cup cream cheese
- ½ teaspoon chili powder
- ½ teaspoon cumin, ground
- ½ teaspoon garlic powder
- Salt and black pepper to the taste

Directions

1. Fill stock in a pot, add cauliflower and onion, heat up over medium heat and cook for 30 minutes. Add chili powder, salt, pepper, cumin and garlic powder and stir.
2. Mix in cream cheese and stir a bit until it melts. Blend using an immersion blender and mix with the mayo. Chill for 2 hours before you serve it. Enjoy!

Nutrition:

40 Calories

1.23g Protein

3.31g Fat

Pesto Crackers

Preparation Time: 10 minutes

Cooking Time: 17 minutes

Servings: 6

Ingredients

- ½ teaspoon baking powder
- Salt and black pepper to the taste
- 1 and ¼ cups almond flour
- ¼ teaspoon basil, dried
- 1 garlic clove, minced
- 2 tablespoons basil pesto
- A pinch of cayenne pepper
- 3 tablespoons ghee

Directions

1. Incorporate salt, pepper, baking powder and almond flour. Whisk garlic, cayenne and basil then pesto.
2. Stir in ghee and mix your dough with your finger. Roll out dough on a lined baking sheet, introduce in the oven at 325 degrees Fahrenheit and bake for 17 minutes.
3. Put aside to cool down, slice crackers and serve them as a snack. Enjoy!

Nutrition:

9 Calories

0.41g Protein

0.14g Fat

Portobello Mushroom Pizza

Preparation Time: 15 minutes

Cooking Time: 5 minutes

Servings: 4

Ingredients:

- 4 large Portobello mushrooms, stems removed
- ¼ cup olive oil
- 1 teaspoon minced garlic
- 1 medium tomato, cut into 4 slices
- 2 teaspoons chopped fresh basil
- 1 cup shredded mozzarella cheese

Directions:

1. Preheat the oven to broil. Line a baking sheet with aluminum foil and set aside. In a small bowl, toss the mushroom caps with the olive oil until well coated. Use your fingertips to rub the oil in without breaking the mushrooms.

2. Place the mushrooms on the baking sheet gill-side down and broil the mushrooms until they are tender on the tops, about 2 minutes. Flip the mushrooms over and broil 1 minute more.

3. Take the baking sheet out and spread the garlic over each mushroom, top each with a tomato slice, sprinkle with the basil, and top with the

cheese. Broil the mushrooms until the cheese is melted and bubbly, about 1 minute. Serve.

Nutrition:

251 Calories

20g Fat

14g Protein

3g Fiber

Garlicky Green Beans

Preparation Time: 10 minutes

Cooking Time: 10 minutes

Servings: 4

Ingredients:

- 1-pound green beans, stemmed
- 2 tablespoons olive oil
- 1 teaspoon minced garlic
- Sea salt
- Freshly ground black pepper
- ¼ cup freshly grated Parmesan cheese

Directions:

1. Preheat the oven to 425°F. Line a baking sheet with aluminum foil and set aside. In a large bowl, toss together the green beans, olive oil, and garlic until well mixed. Season the beans lightly with salt and pepper.

2. Spread the beans on the baking sheet and roast them until they are tender and lightly browned, stirring them once, about 10 minutes. Serve topped with the Parmesan cheese.

Nutrition:

104 Calories

9g Fat

4g Protein

1g Fiber

Sautéed Asparagus with Walnuts

Preparation Time: 10 minutes

Cooking Time: 5 minutes

Servings: 4

Ingredients:

- 1½ tablespoons olive oil
- ¾ pound asparagus, woody ends trimmed
- Sea salt
- Freshly ground pepper
- ¼ cup chopped walnuts

Directions:

1. Place a large skillet over medium-high heat and add the olive oil. Sauté the asparagus until the spears are tender and lightly browned, about 5 minutes.
2. Season the asparagus with salt and pepper. Remove the skillet from the heat and toss the asparagus with the walnuts. Serve.

Nutrition:

124 Calories

12g Fat

3g Protein

2g Fiber

Brussels Sprouts Casserole

Preparation Time: 15 minutes

Cooking Time: 30 minutes

Servings: 8

Ingredients:

- 8 bacon slices
- 1-pound Brussels sprouts, blanched for 10 minutes and cut into quarters
- 1 cup shredded Swiss cheese, divided
- ¾ cup heavy (whipping) cream

Directions:

1. Preheat the oven to 400°F. Place a skillet over medium-high heat and cook the bacon until it is crispy, about 6 minutes. Reserve 1 tablespoon of bacon fat to grease the casserole dish and roughly chop the cooked bacon.

2. Lightly oil a casserole dish with the reserved bacon fat and set aside. In a medium bowl, toss the Brussels sprouts with the chopped bacon and ½ cup of cheese and transfer the mixture to the casserole dish.

3. Pour the heavy cream over the Brussels sprouts and top the casserole with the remaining ½ cup of cheese. Bake until the cheese is melted and

lightly browned and the vegetables are heated through, about 20 minutes. Serve.

Nutrition:

299 Calories

11g Fat

12g Protein

3g Fiber

Creamed Spinach

Preparation Time: 10 minutes

Cooking Time: 30 minutes

Servings: 4

Ingredients:

- 1 tablespoon butter
- ½ sweet onion, very thinly sliced
- 4 cups spinach, stemmed and thoroughly washed
- ¾ cup heavy (whipping) cream
- ¼ cup Herbed Chicken Stock
- Pinch sea salt
- Pinch freshly ground black pepper
- Pinch ground nutmeg

Directions:

1. In a large skillet over medium heat, add the butter. Sauté the onion until it is lightly caramelized, about 5 minutes. Stir in the spinach, heavy cream, chicken stock, salt, pepper, and nutmeg.
2. Sauté until the spinach is wilted, about 5 minutes. Continue cooking the spinach until it is tender and the sauce is thickened, about 15 minutes. Serve immediately.

Nutrition:

195 Calories

20g Fat

3g Protein

2g Fiber

Mini Parsnip Pancakes

Preparation Time: 15 minutes

Cooking Time: 24 minutes

Servings: 4

Ingredients:

- 1 parsnip
- 1 small white onion
- ¼ tsp. nutmeg powder
- 2 eggs
- 1 cup (227 g) almond flour
- 1 cup (227 g) grated cheddar cheese

Directions:

1. Mix the parsnip, onions, nutmeg powder, salt, black pepper, eggs, almond flour, and Monterey Jack cheese. Heat the avocado oil over medium heat.

2. Working in batches, use a scoop to add drops of the mixture into the skillet with intervals. Press down to form patties and fry on both sides for 4 minutes per side. Serve.

Nutrition:

784 Calories

79.88g Fat

1.7g Fiber

Creamy Mashed Cauliflower

Preparation Time: 15 minutes

Cooking Time: 12 minutes

Servings: 4

Ingredients:

- 2 (236 g) head cauliflowers
- 1 cup (227 g) almond milk
- 1/3 cup (74 g) heavy cream
- 4 garlic cloves
- ¼ tsp. nutmeg powder
- 4 tbsp. unsalted butter, room temperature
- 2 tbsp. cream cheese
- 1 tbsp. chopped fresh scallions

Directions:

1. Boil cauliflower and about 2 cups of salted water over medium heat. Reduce the heat and simmer for 10 minutes. Drain and pour into a bowl.

2. As the cauliflower cooked, pour the almond milk in a pot and add the heavy cream, garlic, nutmeg powder, salt, and black pepper. Warm over medium-low heat for 1 to 2 minutes.

3. Mash the cauliflower until smooth. Add the butter, cream cheese, and pour the warm

almond milk mixture. Mix well and combine with the other ingredients.

4. Garnish with the scallions and serve.

Nutrition:

662 Calories

72.08g Fat

5.02g Carbs

Korean Braised Turnips

Preparation Time: 15 minutes

Cooking Time: 27 minutes

Servings: 4

Ingredients:

- 1 large turnip
- 2 tbsp. almond oil
- 2 garlic cloves
- 6 tbsp. coconut aminos
- 3 tbsp. swerve brown sugar
- ½ cup (125 ml) vegetable broth
- 1 cup grated Gruyere cheese

Directions:

1. Boil turnip to a pot and cover with slightly salted water for 5 minutes. Drain.
2. Heat the almond oil in a deep skillet and sauté the garlic until fragrant.
3. Mix the coconut aminos and swerve brown sugar.
4. Toss the turnips in the peanut oil and pour on the coconut aminos mixture. Sauté for 1 minute and add the vegetable broth. Stir well and cook for 20 minutes.

5. Top with the Gruyere cheese and garnish with the peanuts.

Nutrition:

182 Calories

15.57g Fat

0.6g Fiber

Garlic Sautéed Rapini

Preparation Time: 10 minutes

Cooking Time: 11 minutes

Servings: 4

Ingredients:

- 2 tbsp. avocado oil
- 4 garlic cloves
- 2 cups (454 g) rapini

For topping

- 1 cup (227 g) grated Monterey Jack cheese
- 2 tbsp. toasted almond flakes

Directions:

1. Sauté garlic and avocado oil in a large skillet. Mix in the rapini and cook for 10 minutes. Season with salt.
2. Dish onto serving plates, top with the Monterey Jack cheese, almonds, and serve.

Nutrition:

254 Calories

23.91g Fat

0.6g Fiber

Broccoli Fried Cheese

Preparation Time: 15 minutes

Cooking Time: 14 minutes

Serves: 4

Ingredients:

- 1 (225 g) head broccoli
- 2 eggs
- 1 cup (227 g) grated cheddar cheese
- 1/3 cup (74 g) grated Monterey Jack cheese
- 2 tbsp. butter

Directions:

1. Steam broccoli for 10 minutes. Pour the broccoli into a bowl and let cool. Crack on the eggs and mix with the cheeses.
2. Working the batches, melt the butter in a large skillet and fry the broccoli on both sides for 4 minutes per side. Remove the broccoli to a plate and serve warm.

Nutrition:

240 Calories

20.7g Fat

0.3g Fiber

Spicy Butter Baked Asparagus

Preparation Time: 15 minutes

Cooking Time: 15 minutes

Servings: 4

Ingredients:

- ½ lb. (227 g) asparagus
- ½ cup (113 g) salted butter
- 1 tsp. cayenne pepper
- 1 cup grated Monterey Jack cheese

Direction:

1. Ready the oven to 425°F/220°C. Spread the asparagus on a baking tray. Mix the butter, cayenne pepper, salt, and black pepper. Drizzle the mixture on the asparagus and toss well with a spatula. Scatter the Monterey Jack cheese on top.
2. Bake for 15 minutes. Serve afterwards.

Nutrition:

253 Calories

24g Fat

1.3g Fiber

Grilled Zucchini with Pecan Gremolata

Preparation Time: 45 minutes

Cooking Time: 8 minutes

Servings: 4

Ingredients:

- 2 zucchinis
- 4 tbsp. sugar-free maple syrup
- ½ cup (113 g) olive oil
- 2 scallions
- 8 garlic cloves
- 1 cup (227 g) toasted pecans
- 8 tbsp. pork rinds
- 2 tbsp. chopped fresh parsley
- 1 tbsp. plain vinegar

Directions:

1. Sprinkle the zucchinis with salt and let sit for 30 minutes to release liquid. Pat dry with a paper towel. Mix 2 tablespoons oil with the maple syrup and toss with the zucchinis.

2. Heat a grill pan over medium heat and grill the zucchinis for 4 minutes per side. Put in serving platter.

3. Mix the remaining olive oil, scallions, garlic, pecans, pork rinds, parsley, and vinegar. Spoon the gremolata all over the zucchinis and enjoy!

Nutrition:

852 Calories

84.1g Fat

1.4g Fiber

Coconut Cauli Fried Rice

Preparation Time: 10 minutes

Cooking Time: 8 minutes

Servings: 4

Ingredients:

- 2 tbsp. coconut oil
- 1 small red bell pepper
- 1 scallion
- 2 garlic cloves
- 4 eggs, beaten
- 1 cup (227 g) cauliflower rice
- 1 tbsp. coconut aminos
- 1 cup grated cheddar cheese

Directions:

1. Melt the coconut oil in wok and stir-fry the bell peppers for 5 minutes.
2. Mix in the scallions, garlic and cook for 30 seconds.
3. Scramble eggs to the wok. Mix in the cauliflower rice and cook for 2 minutes.
4. Stir in the coconut aminos, sesame seeds, and adjust the taste. Simmer for 1 minute and stir in the cheddar cheese. Turn the heat off and serve immediately.

Nutrition:

251 Calories

20.68g Fat

1g Fiber

Wild Garlic Skillet Bread

Preparation Time: 50 minutes

Cooking Time: 25 minutes

Servings: 4

Ingredients:

- 3 ¼ cups almond flour
- ¼ tsp. erythritol
- ¾ tsp. salt
- ¾ oz. agar powder
- 1 cup lukewarm water
- 3/8 cup melted butter
- 1 cup chopped fresh wild garlic

Directions:

1. In a mixer's bowl, using the dough hook, mix the almond flour, erythritol, salt, and agar agar powder. Add the lukewarm water and combine until dough forms.

2. Dust a surface with almond flour, add the dough and knead with your hands until smooth and elastic.

3. Brush a bowl with melted butter, sit in the dough and cover with a damp napkin. Put the bowl on top of your refrigerator and let rise for 1 hour.

4. After, take off the napkin and press the dough with your fist to release the air trapped in the dough. Divide the dough into 12 pieces and re-shape into a ball.
5. Grease an oven-proof skillet with olive oil and arrange the dough rolls in the pan. Cover with a damp napkin and rise for 30 minutes.
6. Take off, brush the top of the dough with olive oil, and sprinkle with the wild garlic leaves and some flaky salt.
7. Prep oven to 400°F/200°C.
8. Situate skillet in the oven and bake 25 minutes.
9. Let cool. Enjoy!

Nutrition:

893 Calories

28.6g Fat

0.7g Fiber

Crispy Roasted Brussels Sprouts and Walnuts

Preparation Time: 15 minutes

Cooking Time: 14 minutes

Servings: 4

Ingredients:

- 3 tbsp. almond oil
- 1/3 lb. (151.3 g) Brussels sprouts
- 2 garlic cloves
- 1 red chili pepper
- 2 sprigs chopped fresh mint
- ¼ cup (59 ml) coconut aminos
- 1 tbsp. xylitol
- 1 tbsp. plain vinegar
- 1 tbsp. toasted sesame seeds
- ½ cup (113 g) chopped toasted walnuts

Directions:

1. Sauté Brussels sprouts and sesame oil in a large skillet for 10 minutes.
2. Stir in the garlic, red chili pepper, and mint leaves for 1 minute.
3. Mix the coconut aminos, xylitol, and vinegar. Fill mixture over the vegetables and toss. Simmer for 2 minutes.
4. Mix in the sesame seeds, walnuts, and season.

Nutrition:

351 Calories

37.7g Fat

3.3g Carbs

Garlic Cheddar Mushrooms

Preparation Time: 10 minutes

Cooking Time: 6 minutes

Servings: 4

Ingredients:

- 3 tbsp. butter
- 3 garlic cloves
- 1 cup sliced cremini mushrooms
- 1 cup grated cheddar cheese

Directions:

1. Cook butter in a skillet and sauté the mushrooms for 5 minutes.
2. Stir in the garlic and cook for 30 seconds.
3. Dish the food onto serving plates, top with the Parmesan cheese and garnish with parsley. Serve.

Nutrition:

199 Calories

18.27g Fat

0.3g Fiber

Mexican Cauli-Rice

Preparation Time: 10 minutes

Cooking Time: 6 minutes

Servings: 4

Ingredients:

- 2 tbsp. butter
- 2 tbsp. almond oil
- ½ tsp. onion flakes
- 3 garlic cloves, minced
- 1 tbsp. unsweetened tomato puree
- 1 cup (227 g) cauliflower rice
- 1 cup grated Mexican cheese blend
- 2 tbsp. chopped fresh cilantro

Directions:

1. Sauté onion and butter and almond oil in a pot for 30 seconds.
2. Mix in the tomato puree and cook for 2 minutes.
3. Stir in the cauliflower rice, add a quarter cup of water, salt, black pepper, and simmer for 4 minutes.
4. Stir in the Mexican cheese blend afterwards. Garnish with the cilantro and serve warm.

Nutrition:

223 Calories

20.6g Fat

0.7g Fiber

Turnip Latkes with Creamy Avocado Sauce

Preparation Time: 20 minutes

Cooking Time: 16 minutes

Servings: 4

Ingredients:

Turnip Latkes:

- ½ lb. (227 g) turnips
- 1 tbsp. almond flour
- 1 shallot
- 1 egg
- ½ cup (113 g) grated cheddar cheese

Creamy Avocado Sauce:

- ½ avocado
- 1 ½ up (340.5 g) Greek yogurt
- ½ tsp. vinegar
- 1 small garlic clove
- 1 tbsp. avocado oil
- 1 tbsp. chopped fresh cilantro

Directions:

1. Turnip Latkes:
2. Place the turnips in a cheesecloth, fold up and press out as much liquid as possible. Pour the turnips into a bowl and add the almond flour, shallot, egg, cheddar cheese, salt, and black

pepper. Mix well and form 1-inch patties from the mixture.

3. Heat the almond oil in a non-stick skillet over medium heat. Working in batches, add 6 patties and cook for 5 minutes. Cook latkes for 4 minutes

4. Remove the latkes onto a paper towel-lined plate to drain

5. Dill Yogurt Sauce:

6. Mash the avocado. Mix in the Greek yogurt, vinegar, garlic, avocado oil, cilantro, salt, and black pepper.

7. Serve with the avocado sauce.

Nutrition:

518 Calories

51.78g Fat

3.6g Fiber

Cheesy Zucchini Triangles with Garlic Mayo Dip

Preparation Time: 20 minutes

Cooking Time: 30 minutes

Servings: 4

Ingredients:

Garlic Mayo Dip:

- 1 cup crème fraiche
- 1/3 cup mayonnaise
- ¼ tsp. sugar-free maple syrup
- 1 garlic clove
- ½ tsp. vinegar

Cheesy Zucchini Triangles:

- 2 large zucchinis
- 1 egg
- ¼ cup almond flour
- ¼ tsp. paprika powder
- ¾ tsp. dried mixed herbs
- ¼ tsp. swerve sugar
- ½ cup grated mozzarella cheese

Directions:

1. For dip:
2. Mix the crème fraiche, mayonnaise, maple syrup, garlic, vinegar, salt, and black pepper. Wrap with a plastic and chill.

3. Prepare the oven to 400°F and line a baking tray. Set aside.

4. For zucchinis:

5. Put the zucchinis in a cheesecloth and drain. Pour the zucchinis in a bowl.

6. Mix egg, almond flour, paprika, dried mixed herbs, and swerve sugar. Spread the mixture on the baking tray into a round pizza-like piece with 1-inch thickness. Bake for 25 minutes.

7. Reduce the oven's heat to 350°F, take out the tray and sprinkle the zucchini with the mozzarella cheese. Return and bake for 5 minutes.

8. Set aside and then slice the snacks into triangles. Serve with garlic mayo dip.

Nutrition:

401 Calories

41.11g Total Fat

0.2g Fiber

Frozen Strawberry Yogurt Bites

Preparation Time: 90 minutes

Cooking Time: 0 minute

Servings: 10

Ingredients:

- ¼ cup fresh strawberries
- 2 tbsp. sugar-free maple syrup
- ½ tsp. vinegar
- 2 cups Greek yogurt

Directions:

1. Puree strawberries, maple syrup, and vinegar.
2. Spoon the mixture into the holes of an ice-cube tray, halfway up. Top with the Greek yogurt. Spread and freeze for 4 hours.

Nutrition:

106 Calories

10.7g Fat

1g Fiber

Salad Sandwiches

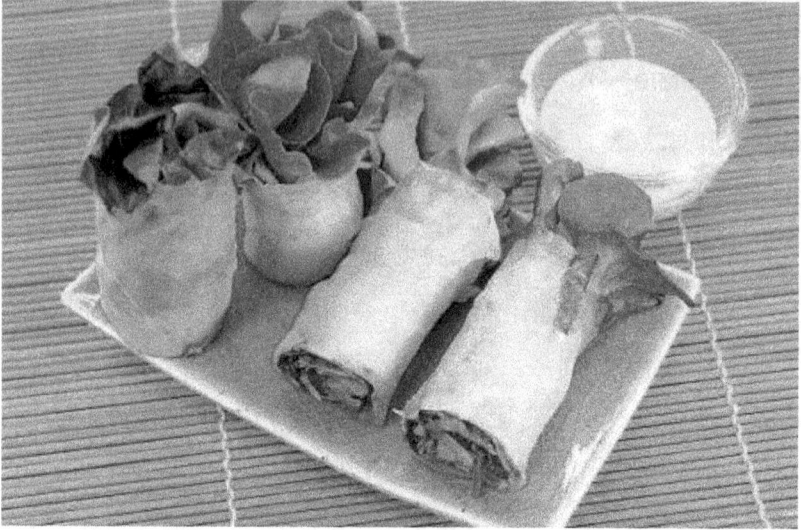

Preparation Time: 5 minutes

Cooking Time: 0 minutes

Servings: 2

Ingredients

1 medium avocado, peeled, pitted, diced.

2 leaves of iceberg lettuce

1-ounce unsalted butter

2-ounce cheddar cheese, sliced.

Directions:

Rinse the lettuce leaves, pat dry with a paper towel, and then smear each leaf with butter.

Top lettuce with cheese and avocado and Serve and enjoy!

Nutrition:

Calories: 187g

Fats: 17 g

Protein: 5 g

Net Carb: 4 g

Fiber: 1.5 g

Celeriac Stuffed Avocado

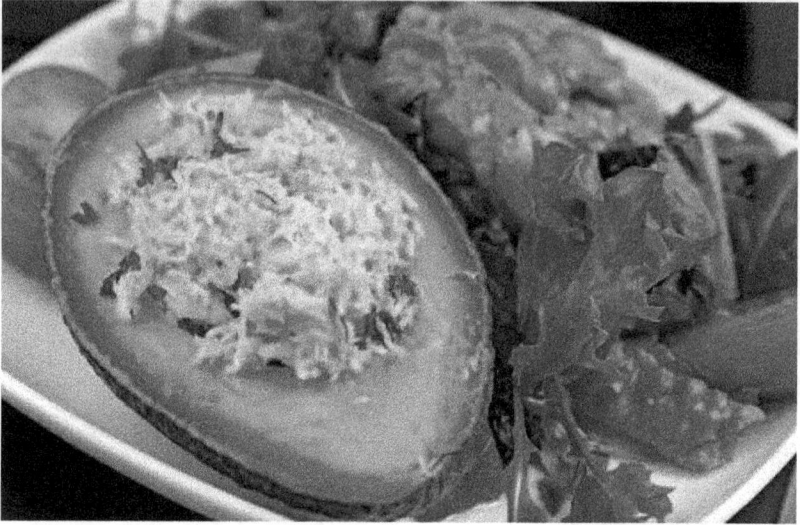

Preparation Time: 10 minutes

Cooking Time: 0 minutes

Servings: 2

Ingredients

1 avocado

1 celery root finely chopped.

2 tbsp. mayonnaise

½ of a lemon, juiced, zested.

2 tbsp. mayonnaise

Others:

¼ tsp. salt

Directions:

Prepare avocado and for this, cut avocado in half and then remove its pit.

Place remaining ingredients in a bowl, stir well until combined and evenly stuff this mixture into avocado halves.

Serve and enjoy!

Nutrition:

Calories: 285

Fats: 27 g

Protein: 2.8 g

Net Carb: 4.4 g

Fiber: 2.6 g

Cobb salad

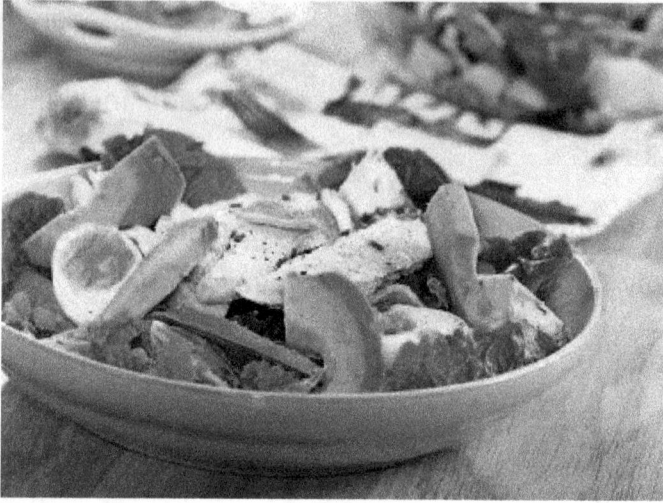

Preparation Time: 5 minutes

Cooking Time: 10 minutes

Servings: 1

Ingredients

1 large egg, hard-boiled, peeled, diced.

2 oz. chicken thigh

2 1/2 slices bacon, cooked, crumbled.

½ of a medium avocado, diced.

½ cup chopped lettuce.

Others:

1 cup of water

3 tbsp. apple cider vinegar

1 ½ tbsp. coconut oil

¼ tsp. salt

1/8 tsp. ground black pepper

Directions:

Cook chicken thigh and for this, place chicken thighs in an instant pot, pour in 1 cup water, and shut the pot with a lid.

Cook the chicken for 5 minutes at high pressure, and when done, let the pressure release naturally.

Meanwhile, cook the bacon and for this, take a skillet pan, place it over medium heat and when hot, add bacon slices.

Cook the bacon for 3 to 5 minutes until golden brown, then transfer them to a cutting board and chop the bacon, reserve the bacon grease in the pan for the next meal.

When chicken thigh has cooked, transfer it to a bowl and shred the chicken with two forks, reserving the chicken broth for later use.

Assemble the salad and for this, place lettuce in a salad plate, top with chicken, bacon, diced eggs, avocado, and chicken in horizontal rows.

Prepare the dressing and for this, whisk together salt, black pepper, vinegar, and oil until incorporated and then drizzle the dressing generously over the salad.

Serve and enjoy!

Nutrition:

Calories: 206

Fats: 11.8 g

Protein: 19.2 g

Net Carb: 6 g

Fiber: 3 g

Cabbage Hash Browns

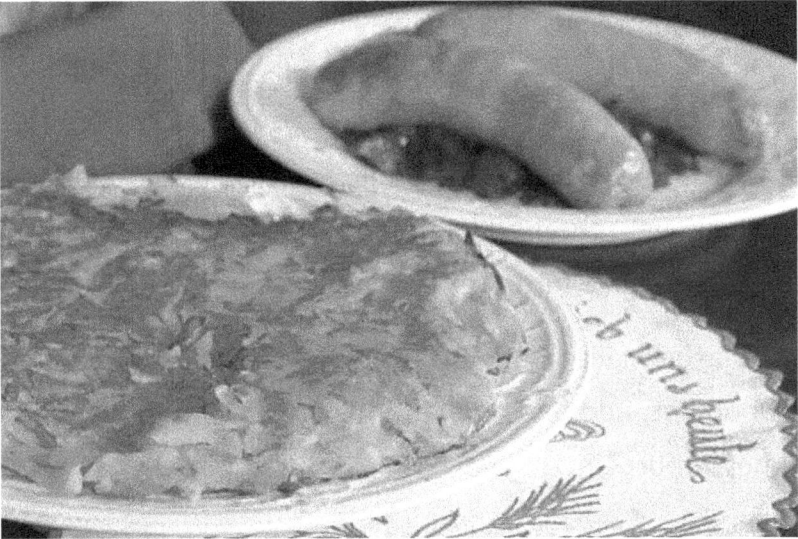

Preparation Time: 10 minutes

Cooking Time: 12 minutes

Servings: 2

Ingredients

1 ½ cup shredded cabbage

2 slices of bacon

1/2 tsp. garlic powder

1 egg

Others:

1 tbsp. coconut oil

½ tsp. salt

1/8 tsp. ground black pepper

Directions:

Crack the egg in a bowl, add garlic powder, black pepper, and salt, whisk well, then add cabbage, toss until well mixed and shape the mixture into four patties.

Take a large skillet pan, place it over medium heat, add oil and when hot, add patties in it and cook for 3 minutes per side until golden brown.

Transfer hash browns to a plate, then add bacon into the pan and cook for 5 minutes until crispy.

Serve hash browns with bacon.

Nutrition:

Calories: 336

Fats: 29.5 g

Protein: 16 g

Net Carb: 0.9 g

Fiber: 0.8 g

Cauliflower Hash Browns

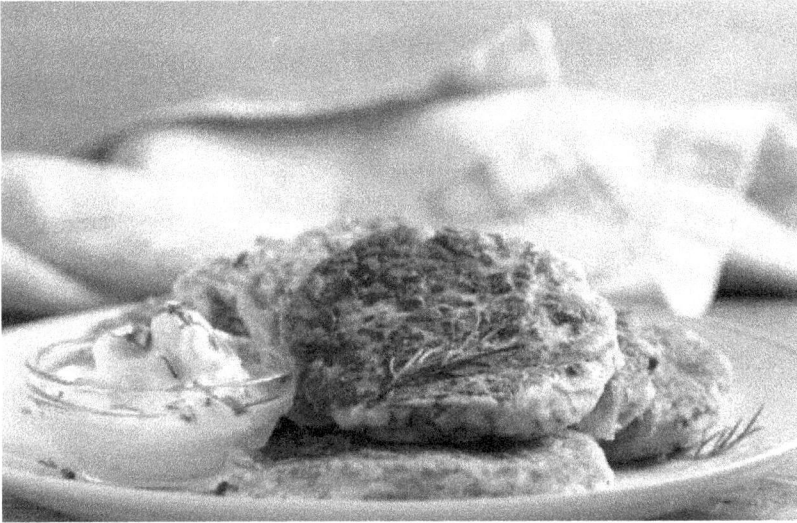

Preparation Time: 10 minutes

Cooking Time: 18 minutes

Servings: 2

Ingredients

¾ cup grated cauliflower

2 slices of bacon

1/2 tsp. garlic powder

1 large egg white

Others:

1 tbsp. coconut oil

½ tsp. salt

1/8 tsp. ground black pepper

Directions:

Place grated cauliflower in a heatproof bowl, cover with plastic wrap, poke some holes in it with a fork and then microwave for 3 minutes until tender.

Let steamed cauliflower cool for 10 minutes, then wrap in a cheesecloth and squeeze well to drain moisture as much as possible.

Crack the egg in a bowl, add garlic powder, black pepper, and salt, whisk well, then add cauliflower, and toss until well mixed and sticky mixture comes together.

Take a large skillet pan, place it over medium heat, add oil and when hot, drop cauliflower mixture on it, press lightly to form hash brown patties, and cook for 3 to 4 minutes per side until browned.

Transfer hash browns to a plate, then add bacon into the pan and cook for 5 minutes until crispy.

Serve hash browns with bacon.

Nutrition:

Calories: 347.8

Fats: 31 g

Protein: 15.6 g

Net Carb: 1.2 g

Fiber: 0.5 g

www.ingramcontent.com/pod-product-compliance
Lightning Source LLC
Chambersburg PA
CBHW050219270326
41914CB00003BA/488